Binge Eating Disorder Treatment

How to Overcome Binge Eating Without Professional Help (Life-Changing Tips and Strategy)

By

Erika Robinson

Table of Contents

Introduction

Binge eating disorder, in brief BED, is a life-threatening condition characterized by frequent incidences of eating huge amounts of food quickly to the state of exhaustion and discomfort.

A person with this disorder frequently has the urge to consume large amounts of foods within a short time, and he/she feels unable to stop. It's like a compulsion that cannot be resisted.

Most people who have this disorder don't have control over the amount of food they eat at a given time. After binge eating, they feel guilty, shame, distress, and unhappy.

To eliminate this guilt or bad feeling, some of them resort to damaging measures to compensate, one of which is purging, just to counteract their binge eating.

This is the most common eating disorder we have in the United States of America. It can occur at any age, but it is most common in the late teens to one's early twenties, and it can last for many years because it is a chronic disease.

Binge eating disorder is seen more in women than men, and it is the most common eating disorder prevalent among men.

Symptoms of Binge Eating

The ciphers and symptoms of binge eating disorder can be both physical and emotional.

The physical signs and symptoms of binge eating are:

- Weight fluctuations
- Stomach cramps, acid reflux, constipation, and other gastrointestinal complaints

The emotional signs of binge eating are:

- Big quantities of food will be missing in a short period
- You will find lots of empty food wrappers and food containers in hidden corners of the home; this indicates a person is consuming a large amount of foods
- Fear of eating with people in public or eating alone in public
- Always practicing new diets
- Hoarding or stealing foods in unusual places
- They create rituals or lifestyles just to make time for binge eating
- They withdraw from their usual hobbies, activities, and friends
- They eat frequently
- Extremely conscious of the shape and weight of their bodies

- Always checking the mirror for flaws in their bodies and appearance
- They eat discretely in a particular period a large amount of food that an individual shouldn't be able to finish at a time.
- They feel totally helpless when trying to stop eating
- Abnormal eating behaviors, e.g., they can eat throughout the day without planning mealtimes, they can skip meals or eat small portions of food during regular meals.
- They develop and take part in food rituals, e.g., they eat only a particular food or food group, and they chew excessively.
- They eat alone because they are trying to avoid embarrassment

- After overeating, they usually feel guilty, disgusted, embarrassed, or depressed
- They have very low self-esteem

Causes of Binge Eating Disorder

Genetics: Eating disorders may run in some families genetically. You can have higher risks of binge eating disorder if any of your parents, grandparents, or great grandparents had it. Studies have even shown that there are some genes that affect eating behaviors, and these genes can be passed on to one's offspring.

These genes act by affecting the circuits in the brain that control mood and appetite. A problem with these genes will escalate your probabilities of having binge eating disorder.

Family: People can learn bad habits from their home and family; it's possible for someone to develop this disorder just by watching their mom or dad overeat. This influence can follow them into adulthood.

Low Self-Esteem: People who are not happy with how they look or people who had a bad notion regarding their body shape have higher risks of coming down with this eating disorder than those who don't.

They usually compare themselves with all these thin models they see on the TV and fashion magazines. This makes them hate their bodies; this leads to low self-esteem, which will definitely lead to binge eating.

The feeling of guilt and shame that they have after binge eating can lead to more overeating.

Strict Dieting: In an effort to lose weight, persons with binge eating disorder start following a strict and unhealthy eating pattern or diets just to lose weight. They can skip meals or eat too little, and when they don't gain weight, they become frustrated and eat more.

Depression: Depression can lead people into binging. Half of the people with this eating disorder suffer from depression but till date, scientists are yet to find out if this eating disorder causes depression or depression causes binge eating.

Some health experts are of the opinion that the guilt and shame they feel after overeating can lead to depression.

Anxiety and Stress: The chance of binging is higher after one has gone through a stressful day or is anxious.

Why You Need to Treat Binge Eating
Binge eating disorder is treatable and should be treated because it affects every organ and system of your body. The earlier it is treated, the greater the chances of recovery and improved health, physically and emotionally.

Another reason why binge eating has to be treated is that it leads to poor quality of life. It contributes to difficulty functioning at work, home, in your personal activities and hobbies, and even social life.

It makes one socially isolated and leads to obesity, the risks factor for many chronic diseases. It also leads to type II diabetes, heart disease, joint problems, sleep disorders, and Gastroesophageal reflux disease (GERD).

Some psychiatric and mental disorders have been linked to binge eating disorder, and some of them are substance abuse, anxiety, bipolar disorder, mood swings, and depression.

Treatment Options

Binge eating disorder is completely treatable and preventable. With fast and proper treatment, most people usually get better and recover. Below are some of the ways binge eating disorder is treated conventionally.

1. Self-help Programmes: This is the major step in the direction of recovery. There are many different programs, you just have to pick the one that suits you, and this should be done under the supervision of a medical doctor or by his recommendations.

There are also self-help books you can get from libraries or online libraries. They contain vital information that can help you overcome this condition. You might also be referred to mental health experts for help.

They might give you a self-help workbook, and you will go through it under their supervision. This is known as "guided self-help." Some people just went through this self-help program alone and recovered from this eating disorder.

2. Pharmacotherapy: In this treatment method, pharmaceutical drugs are given to patients with binge eating disorder to help treat the underlying mental health problem behind this condition.

These medications, in conjunction with other psychiatric treatment, help to improve depression, reduce the binge episodes, and help you gain control of yourself and your appetite.

3. Psychological Therapy: This remedy helps in attacking the root cause or the underlying problems making you to binge eat. This therapy is grouped into three, and they are:

i. Interpersonal Therapy (IPT): This type focuses more on the relationship and social issues and how this can be affecting your eating habits.

ii. Dialectical Behavior Therapy (DBT): This therapy helps and teaches you how to control your emotions.

iii. Cognitive Behavioral Therapy (CBT): This is specially adapted for treating binge eating disorders, in this method, you will talk to a therapist, and he/she will help to introduce new ways of eating, feeling, and thinking about situations.

Psychological therapies are very effective-- they have helped a lot of people overcome binge eating, although some people say the results are not long-lasting.

There have been reports of remission and relapses, especially at the beginning of the treatment.

4. Lisdexamfetamine dimesylate: Also known as Vyvanse, this is the first drug approved by the FDA for treating binge eating disorders in adults. Though quite effective, it is stimulating and addictive.

It has some undesirable side effects like difficulty sleeping, anxiety, increased heart rate, dry mouth, and constipation, amongst other more severe side effects.

It shouldn't be taken for weight loss, and it shouldn't be taken with monoamine oxidase inhibitor, an anti-depressant.

5. Selective Serotonin Reuptake Inhibitors (SSRIs): This is an anti-depressant drug prescribed for people with binge eating disorder. This can be done in addition to the self-help program or without the self-help program.

This drug increases the serotonin in the bran-- this is the chemical messenger in charge of happiness, and it lifts your mood and makes you feel good. This drug can lead to an improvement in your eating habit, but the drawback is that it has some unpleasant side effects.

Some of the side effects of this drug are: low sex drive, anxious, feeling shaky or agitated, insomnia or feeling sleepy, feeling weak or sick, blurred vision, indigestion, and digestive problems, dizziness, constipation or diarrhea, weight loss, and loss of appetite.

Sometimes, these side effects reduce after some times while in others, they persist.

6. Anticonvulsant: Commonly known as Topamax or Topiramate, this migraine prescription drug helps reduce the episodes of binge eating. It is also effective but has a lot of uninvited side effects.

Some of the side effects are kidney stones, high body temperature, eye problems, dizziness, confusion, and suicidal thoughts. There are more serious side effects that can still take place.

Pregnant women or women who are planning to take-in should avoid this drug because it can affect the fetus.

7. Behavioral Weight Loss Therapy: This therapy help people lose weight and reduce the behaviors or signs of binge eating by improving the body image of the patient and his or her poise or self-esteem.

This method of treatment helps the patient to make gradual, healthy changes in lifestyle like diet, thinking pattern, food intake, thoughts about food, and exercise. It also reduces the health complications caused by obesity.

Though this therapy is said to help people lose moderate weight, it mostly brings about short-term recovery, and is not as effective as psychological therapies. It is still worth your try, since different therapies have different level of effect on different individuals. It is also a good alternative for individuals who other therapies were not successful and who are just focused mainly on losing weight.

8. Nutritional Counseling: Individuals with binge eating disorder can go through special nutritional counseling; this will help the patient plan and follow a healthy diet. An exercise routine can also be added, but this will be done under the supervision of a medical doctor or a trained therapist.

This will help you find the triggers of this binge eating disorder, fight malnutrition, nutritional deficiencies, and also make sure you meet the nutritional needs of your brain, major organs, and body.

Eating disorder experts believe that this program should only be carried out if the patient is able to control this eating disorder; else it will definitely trigger it and exacerbate the eating disorder.

Natural Remedies for Binge Eating
1. Reduce Stress

Many health experts agree that stress is one of the underlying health issues contributing to this binge eating disorder. Stress shoves many into eating "comfort food."

People with binge eating disorder should learn how to manage stress effectively; this will enhance long-term recovery and improve their general health.

Learn and practice several ways to soothe yourself and relieve stress, some of the options to try are meditation, regular exercise, spending time with people, listening to music, writing, walking in nature, spending time with nature, reading, playing with pets and having them around, and creating fun hobbies for yourself.

Choose the one or the ones that work best for you and stick with it.

2. Get Help/Support

Open up to loved ones and the people you trust; this is very important in overcoming binge eating disorder and other eating disorders. Studies have shown that opening up and being honest help in making a lot of differences and boosting your chances of recovery.

You can even join a support group, it can be online or offline, or you can call an eating disorder helpline.

3. Proper Hydration

A healthy intake of water can help you overcome this disorder; it improves your mental functions thereby relieving the mental symptoms of binge eating disorder such as agoraphobia and depression.

It helps the body control appetite and food intake; it gets into every cell of your body and ensures that it works well. Electrolytes also require water to work well.

Drink lots of water daily, increase your intake of water during hot weather and after a session of strenuous physical activities or hard labor.

4. B Vitamins

This helps in improving your mood and fights the urge to binge by increasing your levels of serotonin; this will decrease your episodes of binging and assist you to overcome the condition.

5. Manganese

This essential mineral helps in the metabolism and transportation of glucose in the body; it also helps in reducing sugar cravings, which can push one to binge eat.

Manganese also helps to stabilize the concentration of sugar in the bloodstream. Take 10 mg of manganese daily.

6. Zinc

Zinc helps to regulate appetite and control overeating. Take 15 mg every day.

7. L-Glutamine

This supplement helps to stop strong sugar cravings. You can get this supplement in the form of powder or capsules; it also improves your mental functions and clears mental symptoms of binge eating disorder.

Your body converts this supplement into food for your brain. When you have a strong sugar craving, take 500 mg of this supplement, or open the capsules and put the powder on the tongue.

8. 5-HTP

Take this supplement in the evening, or whenever you have the urge to binge eat, it stops the cravings and helps you to control your appetite. It is a precursor to serotonin. It relaxes you and suppresses your appetite.

It also fights anxiety and stress. Take 200 mg daily.

9. Magnesium Glycinate

This supplement calms your brain and improves your mental functions. It also calms your body and stabilizes the levels of glucose in your bloodstream.

The levels of glucose in the body fluctuate greatly when a person has binge eating disorder; this supplement will increase the levels of magnesium in your body and stop this craving.

It also helps one to sleep late at night and also regulates appetite. Take 500 mg every evening.

10. Chromium

This vital mineral helps in reducing the urge to binge, and it also calms your cravings for sugar. It helps to transport insulin into your cells, thereby helping in the regulation of glucose.

When this is done, your body will not be able to send messages to your brain that you need sugar. Take quality chromium supplements, 200 mcg daily.

11. Ashwagandha

This is a powerful adaptogen, it helps relieve stress and anxiety, and it calms your body. It helps you sleep better and boost your immune functions.

12. Kava Kava

This herb calms your body and relieves anxiety; it also relieves insomnia, stress, muscle tension, and spasms. It induces deep sleep and relieves pains.

13. Inositol

This supplement is very helpful in treating moodiness and mood swings, anxiety, depression, and stress. It stops binge eating and sugar cravings, and it also balances the levels of hormones in the body.

14. Gotu Kola

This powerful herb has been used in treating a lot of health problems for over 2000 years. It has powerful mental health benefits. It helps in erasing the mental symptoms of binge eating disorder.

15. Probiotics

These are friendly micro-organisms in your gut and intestinal flora. They improve your appetite and your immune system. They help the procedure of digestion and absorption of nutrients in the body.

When the levels of these healthy bacteria reduce, it will cause a negative change in your body. It will also affect your weight, your appetite, and even your mental functions.

Eat more of fermented food and yogurt-- they are rich sources of probiotics.

16. Digestive Enzymes

This helps the digestion of food and fight malnutrition, which can worsen this condition. It helps your brain get enough nutrients it needs, thereby preventing and improving the mental symptoms of binge eating disorder.

17. Epsom Salt Bath

Before you go to bed, have a hot bath with Epsom salt for 20 minutes, this will relieve anxiety and help you relax well. This salt contains magnesium, a natural stress reliever. It helps you sleep like a little child. Besides, hot water has a good therapeutic effect on the body.

18. Prebiotics

Prebiotics help fight depression and anxiety. They serve as food for the healthy bacteria in your gut, thereby helping them to multiply and do well. These healthy bacteria affect your brain chemistry and help improve your mental performance.

19. Relora

This relieves stress and stops overeating due to stress.

20. Fermented Cod Liver Oil

This helps to relieve the mental symptoms of binge eating disorder like stress, anxiety, and depression. It also reinforces and protects your immune system.

21. Folate

This important B vitamin improves mental performance and helps in the production of chemical messengers like norepinephrine, dopamine, and serotonin.

A low level of this vitamin in the body is linked to depression, moodiness, and other mental problems. The higher the deficiency, the more severe the depression.

Studies have also shown that depressed individuals with low levels of folate do not respond well to antidepressant medications and treatment, and they are susceptible to frequent relapses than others.

Increase your intake of folate-rich foods to help you overcome depression, one of the major symptoms of binge eating disorder. You can meet a doctor to prescribe a good supplement for you.

22. Curcumin

Curcumin is the main active compound in turmeric. It is a potent antioxidant, anti-inflammatory agent, and antidepressant. It fights depression without any unwanted side effects, and it is also a strong remedy for obesity.

It reduces the concentration of cholesterol in the bloodstream, and help one control appetite, especially in those having problem incorporating healthy diet. It helps regain appetite and prevent weight gain at the same time.

The most important effect of Curcumin on binge eating disorder is weight control, appetite control, and relieving depression. You can take turmeric tea or get Curcumin supplement from a good health store.

23. Saffron Extract

This herbal extract helps to retain serotonin in the brain for a longer time. This mood-lifting neurotransmitter helps in fighting moodiness, depression, anxiety, and other mental symptoms associated with this binge eating disorder.

It also treats inflammation and a lot of disorders of the nervous system, it is a powerful antioxidant, and it has many anti-depressant properties. Depression induces binge eating, and this herb combats that.

24. Dopamine Boosters

Dopamine is a neurotransmitter that makes you happy and gives you motivation. This drug is injected into your body intravenously so that it can easily get to the brain.

This helps in controlling moodiness, anxiety, depression, and stress.

25. Ginkgo Biloba

This powerful herb is potent in treating brain-related problems and disorders like anxiety, moodiness, depression, and even binge eating disorder. You can find the capsule or powder in good health stores.

26. Green Tea

Green tea is very rich in an amino acid called L-theanine. This compound helps improve your mood and boost the levels of dopamine, thus fighting the symptoms of binge eating disorder.

27. Phosphatidylserine

This is a supplement that helps improve learning, concentration, memory, and more importantly, the levels of dopamine in the body. It is also used in treating ADHD.

You can get it naturally by eating chicken hearts and cow brains. It also relieves stress by reducing the concentration of stress hormone, cortisol.

28. St. John's Wort

This potent herb has been proven to help treat mild to moderate depression, but it can't treat severe depression. Its anti-depressant property makes it useful in treating the symptoms of binge eating disorder.

It also increases the levels of serotonin in your body. By boosting the levels of this neurotransmitter, it helps to relieve stress, depression, and anxiety.

Serotonin controls your mood, appetite, memory, sleep, learning, and concentration. Do not take this herb with prescription drugs and drugs that treat this eating disorder because they can interact and cause complications in your body.

Let your doctor know if you are taking this herb or supplement before he prescribes drugs for you.

29. Gymnema

This is a traditional herb used in treating diabetes in Ayurveda medicine. Its name in Hindi means "destroyer of sugar," it has a powerful anti-diabetic property, and it is used in eating disorder treatment to relieve sugar cravings.

It also diminishes the hazards of diabetes, one of the health impediments caused by binge eating disorder. You can chew on the fresh leaves or get the tea from a good health store.

When you chew the leaves, it interferes with the ability of your tongue to taste sweet things. It delays the absorption of glucose and fill your taste buds' receptors for sweet taste. It also blocks sugar-binding sites in the body and prevents the accumulation of sugar molecules in the body.

30. Essential Fatty Acids

These fatty acids must be gotten through the foods you eat because the body can't manufacture them. They support the growth, development, and functions of your brain. They also enhance nerve functions and regulate body metabolism.

Low concentrations of these essential fatty acids lead to depression, aggressiveness, and suicidal thoughts. You can get these fatty acids from flaxseeds, flax oil, oily fish, fish oil, grains, and vegetable oils.

You can get quality supplements at a good health store.

31. Increase your Intake of Proteins

Protein-rich food help keep you feeling full for a long time-- this will help regulate your food intake and appetite. It also fights obesity by reducing your body weight and your fat mass. It helps to decrease your daily calorie intake by 441 calories.

High protein diet also improves your metabolism, and it raises the levels of the hormone that helps in suppressing appetite, GLP-1. Rich sources of proteins are legumes, seeds, nuts, fish, meat, and eggs. High protein food also regulates cravings.

32. Don't Skip Breakfast

Yes, you must have heard that breakfast is your most essential meal of the day. That is true, and you should not skip it even if you are trying to lose weight.

Breakfast will help to kick start your metabolism. It will help reduce hunger and cravings, thereby reducing your chances of binge eating later in the day. It will help you on track on your way to recovery. A quality breakfast helps in reducing hunger throughout your day.

To get a more positive effect, make sure your breakfast is protein-rich, it will help to reduce the levels of ghrelin, hunger hormone, and keep you full till it's time to have lunch.

Include fiber-rich foods in your breakfast too-- they also promote fullness and regulate food intake and appetite. Fiber supports healthy functions of your digestive system and prevent some digestive symptoms of binge eating like constipation or diarrhea.

33. Eat Fiber-Rich Food

Increase your intake of food rich in fiber, such as legumes, oatmeal, fruits and vegetables, whole grains, and some herbs. Fiber makes you feel full for a long period thus averting overeating.

It controls hunger, appetite, and regulate food intake. It also cuts cravings and reduces your intake of calories, thus, guiding against obesity, a common complication of binge eating disorder.

Prebiotic fiber serves as food for the healthy bacteria (probiotics) in your gut. They also increase the levels of leptin in the body. This hormone increases satiety and reduces hunger, thus preventing binge eating.

Prebiotic fiber can be found in green leafy vegetables.

34. Get Sufficient Sleep

Insufficient sleep leads to increased appetite, and it has a great impact on hunger levels. Studies have also linked binge eating to insomnia and other forms of sleeplessness.

Short duration of night sleep increases the levels of ghrelin in the body. This is the hormone that signals hunger. Short periods of night sleep also reduce the levels of leptin in the body. This hormone tells your brain that you are full.

Insomnia and sleeping less than 8 hours at night increases body weight and leads to obesity. Try to get sufficient sleep, and it will help you overcome this condition.

Sleep also relaxes your mind, improves your mood, temperament, and relieves stress, anxiety, and depression.

35. SAM-e

This is a powerful natural remedy for depression. It increases the levels of neurotransmitters that control mood, appetite, and memory. It effectively increases the levels of dopamine and serotonin in the body.

This makes you happy, cheerful, and less depressed, thereby relieving the symptoms of binge eating disorder and give you control over yourself.

Health Risks Associated with Binge Eating

There are a lot of health risks and complications caused by binge eating disorder. It affects every part of your body and causes havoc to your vital organs and system. Below are some of the health complications caused by this disorder.

Cardiovascular System: Binge eating and purging make one consumes fewer calories than what the body needs. When this happens, your body has to break down its organs and tissues so it can get fuel for energy.

The first to be broken down are your muscles, and your heart is the most important organ made of muscles. This leads to a slow heartbeat and low blood pressure (hypotension) because the heart is now weak and incapable of pumping blood.

Your blood pressure will continue to get lower and lower, and it also raises your risks of heart failure. When you vomit or make use of laxatives to purge, depletes the levels of electrolytes in your body.

Electrolytes are important chemicals. These include potassium, chloride, and sodium. Potassium helps your heart beat properly, and it also helps in muscle contraction. These electrolytes are barred from the body via purging.

When they are lacking or absent in your body, it leads to heart malfunctions, heart failure, irregular heartbeats, and possibly death. The metabolic rate of the body will also be reduced-- this is an attempt made by the body to conserve energy.

Endocrine System: The hormones that control many processes in your body are made with the cholesterol and fat that you get from food. When you don't get enough of this from the food you eat, the levels of hormones in your body will drop.

The hormones mostly affected are thyroid hormones and sex hormones. Reduced sex hormones cause menstruation problems and infertility. It also causes bone loss (osteoporosis and osteopenia) and also increases the risks of fractures and broken bones.

When binge eating is done over time, your body can become resistant to insulin, and this leads to type II diabetes. Without enough energy, your brain can't regulate temperature, thus leading to a drop in your internal temperature and before you know it, hypothermia may set it.

Starving your body of vital nutrients leads to high levels of cholesterol also.

Digestive System: Restricting your intake of food and purging leads to slow digestion of food known as gastroparesis. It interrupts stomach emptying and leads to many gastrointestinal problems like bloating, stomach pains, bacterial infections, vomiting, nausea, feeling full after eating just a little quantity of food, solid masses of undigested food blocking the intestine, and fluctuations in the levels of blood sugar.

Inadequate intake of vital nutrients such as fiber can lead to constipation. Long-term malnutrition weakens the muscles of your intestines, and they become too weak to expel undigested food from the body.

Abuse of laxatives will damage the nerve endings and can make the body depend on them for proper bowel movement. Binge eating ruptures your stomach and leads to a life-threatening emergency.

Regular vomiting wears down your esophagus-- it tears it and also creates a life-threatening condition. It also causes a hoarse voice and sore throat. Your glands that produce will also get swollen.

Purging and malnutrition raise the risks of pancreatitis-- this is an inflammation of the pancreas, and the major symptoms are vomiting, nausea, and pains. It also leads to intestinal infection, perforation, and obstruction.

Neurological System: One-fifth of the calories you eat go to the brain alone even though it only weighs 3 pounds. Binge eating, dieting, self-starvation, and extreme fasting deprive the brain of these calories, leading to loss of energy.

This manifests in the form of concentration problems, memory problems, and obsessing about foods. Extreme hunger leads to difficulty falling asleep or staying asleep, same with extreme fullness.

Inadequate intake of healthy fats affects the protective layer of lipids covering and insulating the neurons. This leads to tingling and numbness in your hands and feet, including other extreme areas of your body.

Neurons make use of electrolyte to send chemical signals and electric messages to your brain and body, electrolyte imbalance and inadequate intake of water can affect this process and can lead to muscle cramps and seizures.

Malnutrition lessens the volume of blood in the body. This leads to dizziness and fainting, especially when standing. This is more pronounced when enough blood cannot get to the brain.

Obese individuals with binge eating disorder have increased risks of sleep apnea, a condition when one stops breathing while sleeping.

Skin and Hair: Low intake of fats and calories lead to brittle hair, dry skin, and they cause the hair to break and fall. The body grows lanugo (fine, downy hair) in an attempt to conserve warmth during starvation.

Other Consequences: Prolonged and severe dehydration cause kidney failure. Malnutrition decreases the number of blood cells, especially white blood cells which fight diseases.

Fewer amounts of red blood cells in the body or inadequate intake of iron-rich foods can lead to anemia and shortage of blood in the body. Signs of anemia are shortness of breath, weaknesses, dizziness, and fatigue.

Conclusion

Binge eating is completely treatable if you cooperate with your doctor or therapist. While you are undergoing treatment, it is advisable that you forget about losing weight for now because the desire to lose weight pushes one into a restrictive or frequent diet, which in turn leads to binge eating.

Then you have to focus on you as an individual, your personality, character, values, and goals. Your body doesn't define you, your goals, or what you will achieve.

Learn to love your body and improve your self-esteem. Binge eating is seen as a mental problem and treated as such, so work on your mental health and the perception you have about yourself.

Concentrate on your health, and forget about the scale. Focus on how to love your body by eating healthy, nutritious, and well-balanced meals. You can get the help of a nutritionist to help you achieve this and always remember that you are fearfully and wonderfully made.